Secrets of Male Catheter Insertion for Prostate Problems

How to Insert a Catheter Safely and Easily Without Pain

A Manual for Men, Health Practitioners and Students, and Emergency Room Nurses

Ronald M. Bazar

Secrets of Male Catheter Insertion for Prostate Problems

How to Insert a Catheter Safely and Easily Without Pain

A Manual for Men, Health Practitioners and Students, and Emergency Room Nurses

Ronald M. Bazar

Published by:
Ronald M. Bazar, PO Box 73, Cortes Island, BC V0P 1K0
Canada

Email: healthyprostate@ymail.com

First Edition: July 2014

Acknowledgements

I thank Coreen Boucher at Lucent Edits, who again has come to my rescue to make this book as smooth flowing and readable as could be done! (www.lucentedits.com)

Table of Contents

iv

Introduction

The purpose of this book is to help men find a quick solution to an emergency that many men can suddenly face: what to do if you can't pee!

I have been there—10 years ago. I woke up in the middle of the night and had to go something fierce, and not a drop would come out! So I know exactly what this experience is like.

Over the years it happened many times, and I learned how to use a catheter myself. I even got superb advice from expert emergency room nurses who deal with this problem all the time. They taught me some very important techniques that can make catheter insertion easier.

You see, it is very different to insert a catheter when you have a prostate blockage problem versus when you don't have one, but have another reason to use a catheter such as a spinal cord injury or bladder problem.

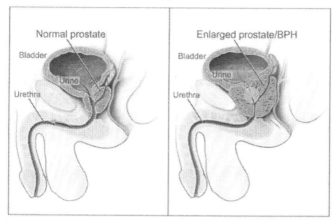

Prostate blockages create their own challenges. The prostate is enlarged or inflamed and very sensitive. This puts pressure on the part of your pee tube—known as the prostatic urethra—that goes right through your prostate. If there is too much pressure, your pee tube will be squeezed closed so tight that not a drop can get through from your bladder no matter how desperately you gotta go.

When something triggers a prostate attack, your prostate can shut you down so that you are unable to pee. With every passing minute, your pain and misery increase because more and more urine is being released into your bladder from your kidneys, but it can't get past your prostate! Thank goodness for the invention of the modern catheter! Without it, a very painful death could happen.

In the old days, a reed was used but I cannot imagine that being easy to do or readily available!

Proper catheter technique then becomes very important so that you can navigate your catheter through the tight passageway created by your enlarged prostate, as it squeezes your pee tube shut.

With the right catheter and technique, let me assure you that insertion is not painful as you would imagine and fear. In fact, discomfort is a more appropriate way to describe it—if it's done properly.

Although the best course of action for you is to visit your emergency room, this book is for those who may have a reoccurring problem or who do not have access to emergency services because they either can't afford it or are too far away from the hospital.

The intent of this guide is not to replace professional medical services but to give you all the hard-earned lessons—which I have gleaned over the years as I faced this painful problem myself—in case you need or want to do it yourself or you are in an emergency and someone has to do it for you.

It also contains some important tips and insights for frontline health practitioners and students and emergency room nurses. If you are one of these people, this book just may help you to succeed in some extreme cases or to make it less traumatic for your patient. You may find an invaluable tip or two throughout the book in addition to the advanced tips for professionals at the end of the book.

I direct most of my language to men who need to do self-catheterization themselves, and I thus provide very detailed procedures. But if you are a practitioner reading this, please do not assume you know it all, as the story I tell later about my urologist's mistake with sanitary practice will make clear.

Most of what is in here, you can find in my guide, *Healthy Prostate: The Extensive Guide to*

Prevent and Heal Prostate Problems, but I have included many new tips in this book. So if you have a problem, this book is well worth the price for what you will learn. You can find the book at this URL: www.healthyprostate.co/

A catheter—and the instructions to use it—should be part of an emergency first aid kit as well as a travel kit.

Imagine you are off in the bush hiking a long way from a hospital, are on the ocean on a boat or a kayak trip, or are on a long flight. Yes, you may be able to get help to come to you but knowing what to do can sure make your life a lot safer and easier than having to wait hour upon hour as the pressure on your bladder builds and builds. No fun, that's for sure. So learn these techniques, and what I call secrets, because they sure are not common knowledge. They just may save you from added misery—or worse.

I sure wish that I had this information years ago. It would have saved me a lot of pain and anguish with my extreme, enlarged prostate condition.

There is a lot to learn but you will become quite knowledgeable fast. When I get into the details of how to do male catheter insertion, I provide every step you need. The reality is that it is quite easy to do once you know how. I want you to know how to precisely execute all the steps and to know the importance of being very sanitary while doing them so that insertion is safe to do yourself.

The thought for most men of passing a tube through the penis triggers anxiety and a very unpleasant reaction of pain and fear. It sure is not the preferred use of the male instrument! I want to assure you that it doesn't have to be like that. Yes, uncomfortable, but not painful like you might imagine.

Once you know what I share with you here, it will be far better than the agony of not peeing at all! And it will not hurt like you may be fearing. You need the right tools and the secrets of how to insert a catheter safely and easily without pain.

What qualifies me to author such a book with no medical degrees or training? You might say it has been my frontline experience as a patient and as a published author specializing in prostate issues with five books on the subject (see list of books on back page). An extremely enlarged prostate with BPH, several prostate crises, and the desire to learn all I could to avoid prostate surgery (which I did) has given me the opportunity to garner what I share in this booklet.

Now let's get to it!

Disclaimer:
This book is for your educational purposes only and not to give you advice about what to

do. If you choose to follow any of the suggestions herein, it is your responsibility in conjunction with your doctor or health practitioner—and not mine. I can take no responsibility for your actions and decisions and much of the material is my opinion for you to examine and learn from as you see fit. You are the boss of your body—not me! Got it? If not, read no further and request a refund.

Chapter 1:
Triggers of Prostate Attacks

Sadly for men, the incidence of prostate disease and problems have skyrocketed over the past decades.

Although many doctors claim the cause of this is aging, the real causes are what we have done to our food and other inputs. These are the causes that I write about extensively in my book *Healthy Prostate: The Extensive Guide to Prevent and Heal Prostate Problems* (www.healthyprostate.co/).

In this section, we'll focus on what I call 'prostate attacks' and their triggers. A prostate attack happens when you experience a sudden surge of prostate symptoms worse than any you have had or when you discover—now, for the first time—symptoms that you never had before, and you realize that you really do have a prostate problem. Ouch! Usually a prostate attack means you are having extreme difficulty urinating or you can't pee at all!

Something actually triggered the sudden shut down. You were having prostate problems— frequent peeing, waking at night, some hesitation when urinating or a burning sensation sometimes when trying to go—but perhaps not serious enough to cause a major problem. Maybe you didn't even think twice about these problems or didn't realize you were having symptoms because they worsen so slowly over time... But now something has happened, and you had a huge reaction that is shutting you down. (That describes me 10 years ago!)

Yikes! You are trying to pee and nada drop to be! And you just gotta go something fierce!

First of all, let's look at what triggers a sudden inability to urinate.

What Triggers the Attack?

In all my prostate attacks, I have always been able to trace the trigger back to something I ate or a supplement or pill I reacted to. It could even be a small amount of something like the wrong vegetable oil, a rancid spice, some mold, or even a trusted food that I began reacting to out of the blue.

Usually the triggers will be something you ate that day (most likely at lunch or supper) or even a new medicine. Most likely, you have consumed something that you are reacting to—sort of an allergic reaction in the prostate.

Avoid medicines that can affect the prostate, such as antihistamines, decongestants and anti-depressants. If you already have an enlarged prostate condition, these drugs can push you over the edge, and you can find yourself in shut-down mode! If you do end up in shut-down mode, look back to the last 24 hours to see if you can remember taking a cold medication or antihistamine, or something else.

Alcohol, especially hard alcohol, and even wine or beer can trigger acute prostate swelling in some men. Limit alcohol to 1–2 drinks per day at most. For some people marijuana can also trigger a prostate attack. Too much of a food, superfood, or supplement (no matter how "good" or "healthy" it is) that you have been eating over time—especially if it contains phytic acid—can trigger an allergic reaction of swelling in the prostate.

Also, if you drank too many liquids before bed, you have added stress to the bladder during the night.

To learn how to personally test for foods or supplements that can cause a reaction in your body please read one of my other books *Healthy Prostate* (www.healthyprostate.co/) or *Prostate Health Diet* (tiny.cc/nu16hx):

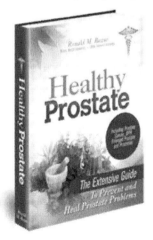 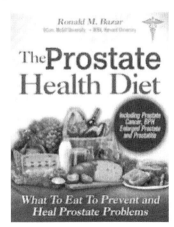

The important thing is to find out what caused your prostate attack so you can avoid it—and hopefully any more—by testing your inputs before they can do you harm.

When I speak about triggers, it does not mean that each time I ate that item it would result in a prostate attack, but at a particular time it did. The items listed below will give you an idea of some of my common triggers:

- too many greens, whether powdered or fresh vegetables; in my case, my own garden kale and super green powders are triggering. I have had a bit too much of them, thinking they were all good! Greens can be hard on the body, so cooked is often better and eaten with butter soothes them, especially if you have a sensitivity to these foods;
- green powders—make sure you test and retest often. I forgot and, woops, blocked one night;
- oils like canola and safflower (now I know better and I avoid these);
- nuts like almonds, cashews, and so on, especially before I learned about phytate reduction by soaking these types of foods;
- sesame seeds;
- unsoaked grains that are quickly cooked;
- chocolate cookies;

- a piece of bagel that I ate, which had a moldy taste; and
- some herbal teas.

These above-mentioned foods are things I have to pay attention to. They may be fine for you, but you will have your own list of foods that can trigger a prostate reaction. As you get healthier, your reactions will reduce. Just remember that a reaction that causes an attack is not your normal state of health. No need to panic and rush for the latest surgeries or interventions.

So be vigilant, find out what your triggers are, **and avoid the culprits** (for now). The triggers will lessen if you make changes to your inputs, and you will find your tolerance to some will come back. You may also learn how to prepare foods in a way that won't cause a reaction.

What to Do When You Have a Prostate Attack

If you wake up and find yourself under a prostate attack or it strikes you suddenly during the day and urination is difficult, painful or impossible—don't panic! There are things you can do, the crisis will pass, and then you can take corrective and preventive action. Try these tips before deciding to use a catheter. Here is what to do. There is a chance that they may work, and you can pee.

Relax and Breathe

If you were awakened, lie down again and try to make your prostate area relax. Sometimes while asleep you force "not peeing" (of course) by not waking up, and this holding back can traumatize your prostate and the bladder sphincter if you are having a reaction to something.

Relaxation can give these parts of your body a chance to reset. By relaxing and breathing, even just a bit, sometimes the spasm or intensity will ease and allow some urine to flow. Don't push as that creates stress in the prostate. Breathe deep and allow some relaxation even if it hurts badly.

It may help to have a plastic pee bottle instead of having to head to the bathroom.

If you can get a little to pass, you may be on your way. Lie down again and repeat. Relax. This process can allow a bit more to come out. Sometimes that is all you need to do and more and more will come out over the next 30 minutes to an hour, and then you should be okay.

Let the waves pass and relax, knowing that letting go and getting all your muscles to loosen up will help. After a minute or two get up, and sit down to pee on the toilet to see if you can release a bit. If you are lucky and something starts to come out, that is a very good sign, even if only a few drops come out (of course you want to let a ton more out!), but getting any amount is a great beginning. It may hurt like hell as you pee, like a burning fire. Try to breathe and relax no matter how painful it is.

Lie down again. Relax, relax and breathe, breathe and relax. Wait and relax. When relaxed and the urge to go comes again, in a minute or two, then again go and see if some more comes out. If lucky, a little more will come out. It is better to sit and relax than to continue standing and trying to pee.

It could take a dozen or more of little pees before you are empty, little by little letting go. Usually the pees will get better and better at some point releasing more. Repeat these steps, but do not go back to sleep until you have a complete empty feeling. It can take an hour or two for you to finally empty your bladder.

If you still have urine in your bladder, avoid going back to sleep. Going back to sleep too soon can cause a further reckoning an hour or two later, and it will be worse if you did not completely empty your bladder. If you drank a lot of liquids in the evening, then staying up a while longer may be wise. This avoids the blocking conditions that often arise while asleep. You may be tired, but once you are flowing, it is best to keep the channels open by staying awake.

Do Not Go Back to Sleep

Get up no matter how tired you feel. I have made the mistake of thinking too soon that the crisis has passed and awoke again an hour or two later with a worse problem.

Know this: The crisis will pass. This is not a normal state of affairs for your prostate. You are having a strong reaction. You can get through it.

Other Helpful Tips

If the above does not work, get a hot water bottle and fill it with the hottest water that you can without burning your skin. Lie down and place it on your pubic bone and lower abdomen/stomach area. A thin towel may help to avoid burning. Relax as much as you can. The heat can have an almost instant effect and can help the relaxing and releasing.

This process may allow some urine to start flowing when you go pee. Keep at it for a few more minutes, giving the heat a chance to penetrate. Pee a bit, lie down with the hot water bottle again, breathe and relax, and soon you will release some more. Once you get a few drops to pass, it often will lead to more, little by little.

If you can have a bowel movement, do so as this will release pressure on the prostate through the thin rectal wall. Even a bit of pressure reduction can make a difference to help the prostate relax and release.

Repeat the hot water bottle application and relax. Hopefully you will experience some opening. Keep calmly saying to yourself, "Relax and release. Relax and release. Relax and release. Breathe deeply, deeply and relax."

You can also massage the perineum area between the scrotum and rectum with some oil, ideally castor oil, while lying down. Try pressing deeply on the spot about 1 inch from the rectum towards the scrotum in the perineum area. This spot is the closest to the prostate. Massage and press that whole area.

Walking may help if lying down doesn't. Try movement and light exercise like sun salutations from yoga. Being vertical may help but could be putting too much downward pressure on the bladder sphincter. You will just have to see what works.

Another method is the sitz bath procedure: 10 minutes with your lower body in hot water with your legs and upper body out of the water. Then do another sitz bath for 2–3 minutes with cold water. You may need to reduce this time to 5 minutes hot and 1 minute cold if the pain is too intense. Repeat once or twice.

Or just use hot and cold compresses to see if that does the trick.

Do not wait too long to try the above techniques. In serious blockages, they just may not work. If you take too long in this stage, more pressure is added to the bladder as the kidneys continuously release more urine. Allow at most 30–60 minutes to get progress, otherwise...

...if nothing works then it is time for a catheter. Heading to the emergency room may be the best option for you at this point. If that is not possible, then you must use the catheter yourself.

Here is one last and very important tip: When you block and have tried some of the suggestions to release and they are not working, it can be best to decide early on to use the catheter rather than wait too long. The longer you wait the more traumatized you and your bladder become, and it can be difficult to follow the steps if you are shaking all over.

Relief is at hand and it is not hard to do. So, decide to use the catheter earlier rather than later if you seem to be so blocked that you are not making any headway. It's a blessing waiting there for you if you need it. Know that your pain of blockage can be gone in minutes by inserting a catheter.

When to Self-Catheterize

The first thing I want to share with you is that using a catheter sounds way worse than it actually is. If you have heard horror stories, then know that it does not have to be like that for you.

In fact, doing it myself was far gentler than when it was done to me by hospital staff! Why? Because you have complete control and, with my tips (that not all emergency room staff know), you can get the job done with only discomfort and much less pain than you feel when the pee can't come out! **A well lubricated catheter tube going through your pee tube does not hurt if done correctly!**

If you have ever had a catheter inserted at a hospital and it was painful, here is why: some hospitals try to save money by using non-lubricated catheters. And then they try to save more by using their equivalent of KY Jelly rather than a superior lubricant that also contains some desensitizer. Also, the catheter they used could have been a diagnostic type, which is much thicker, and could well cause pain especially if not using a desensitizer for insertion.

If you buy the right type and/or the ideal lubricant, and you know how to use it, then the pain is minimal. In fact, it is more a discomfort than a pain. What is painful is the fact that you can't pee and—because of it—you are in distress. In a matter of minutes you can find relief and, oh—what a feeling that is! Believe me!

Do you remember the story of the Spartans at Thermopylae? A small band of elite warriors held off tens of thousands of invading hordes at the pass and saved Greece from takeover. They were able to accomplish this because it is fairly easy to block a pass. Why am I telling you this?

Because the urethra tube that empties your bladder flows through your prostate and even the smallest amount of blockage can shut the pass down completely or weaken the flow to a painful trickle.

I have suffered with benign prostatic hyperplasia, or BPH, and have had the "joy" (joking!) of inserting catheters at least dozens of times. I'll share all of my tips with you.

What is a Male Catheter?

Catheters come in different lengths for males and females and in different thicknesses or gauges (diameters). Thinner ones are used for children and thicker ones for long-term use so that they do not clog with debris or blood clots. A male catheter is longer than a woman's because it has to travel through the penis to get to the bladder, so male catheters are about 12 to 16 inches long.

Sounds scary!

Yes, it does if you have never had one inserted. It is not the favorite use of the male penis, that's for sure! Just the opposite of what you want!

So, for many men, the idea of it is frightening—best to avoid it. Who wants one?? The reality is that they can save your life and make living with a prostate problem much easier. A male catheter can also help you void when you can't and can give you a chance to learn how to heal your prostate.

Prostate enlargement is the leading cause of needing to use a catheter for men. The prostate squeezes the urethra shut and you can't go, no matter how badly you want to!

The pain becomes terrible. You will end up in the emergency ward if you do not know about male catheter insertion.

It is possible to insert it yourself once you know how to avoid catheter problems.

Self-catheterization sounds a lot worse than it is. It does not have to be painful or horrific. In fact, compared to the pain of your bladder filling up and trauma of not knowing how you'll release it, inserting a disposable catheter is nothing.

At the end, when relief finally comes, you'll be thanking this little device.

I was buying catheters at a pharmacy a few years ago, and the pharmacist said he sells many types of catheters these days. This was unheard of before. (My Dad was a pharmacist, and I worked alongside him for years as a teen.

We didn't even have catheters then, only condoms hidden away in a drawer and only to be sold discretely!) Today many, many men are dealing with an enlarged inflamed prostate.

Chapter 2:
Types of Catheters for Men

You'll need to know the types of catheters in the event that all else fails when you are having a prostate attack, and you either can't or don't want to go to emergency. Of course, you will have to prepare in advance so that you have the tools of this trade at hand.

If you do have prostate symptoms and/or are prone to prostate attacks, you should always have a male catheter kit on hand when traveling or at home for emergencies. Doing it yourself is far less stressful than going to emergency rooms and waiting and waiting. Self-catheterization is much easier and less painful than you may imagine.

Obviously, if you do not have a catheter and no urine is coming out, then seeing a doctor or going to the emergency room is the solution. Know that there is no danger of bladder eruption for quite a long period, even up to 24–36 hours. The pain may be extreme, but you have time to get help.

Also, be aware that something triggered the attack. If you can figure it out—now or later—then you will have good information about what not to do again, and you can avoid repeating the experience.

There are several very specialized types of catheters but, for our purposes, there are two versions of catheters for men: internal and external catheters.

- Internal catheter = Stopped. Can't Go.
- External catheter = Going. Can't Stop.

The internal catheters are used to help you pee when your prostate blocks your pee tube.

The external catheters are for opposite conditions: leakage or frequency in which you do not want to have to run (or can't run) to the washroom to pee (e.g., traveling or at a ball game) or if you have a sudden urgency to go that you can't control.

An external catheter is like a condom with a tube at the end that goes to a small bag on your leg. You go when you have to and can empty the bag later. A condom catheter is a very convenient device with no pain and peace of mind. We describe them in detail later.

Here our focus is on the internal catheters because those are the ones we need to use to pee when we're blocked. There are basically two types of internal catheters:

- **single-use** catheters, also known as short-term or intermittent catheters. They are inserted and then removed after you have emptied your bladder, and
- **long-term** catheters, also known as indwelling Foley catheters or just Foley catheters. They have an inflatable balloon function at the end to allow the catheter

to stay inside without slipping out. These are used after surgery or for extreme conditions, such as long-term acute urinary retention.

If you have a sudden prostate block and can't pee, what you want is a simple, single-use, male catheter. You can buy them at your pharmacy, medical supply store, or online (see the sources listed below).

But first let me explain more about these single-use, internal male catheters.

Single-Use, Internal Catheters

Now there are many features you'll want to understand before purchasing a catheter for single-use:

- stiffness
- size and gauge
- lubricated or non-lubricated
- the type of tip for catheter insertion

Stiffness

There are various levels of flexibility: very flexible, medium flex and stiffer. They each have an advantage. The flexible ones are very soft and pliable, which is nice but may be a bit harder to insert all the way through an enlarged prostate, so I rule those out. They are best for long-term usage because of their softness. The stiffer versions can allow an easier transit during the last stage through the prostate and into the bladder. Catheters, by the way, are inexpensive unless you have to use them all the time.

Size and Gauge

Catheters come in different thicknesses called "gauge" and vary from 8 to 28 gauge.

For your emergency use, you want to get 12-gauge or 14-gauge catheters. These are quite thin. Sixteen gauge is important to have as a backup just in case the thinner ones do not work. Boys use 8–10s. They come all the way to 28 gauge (ouch!). Emergency rooms tend to use the 16-gauge ones because they can be made to slide through easier if the prostate really presses your urethra shut.

Lubed or Not Catheters

Both styles work well but lubricated ones, which are ready to use right out of the package, simplify things greatly.

Non-Lubricated Catheters

These types require you to use some kind of lubrication to help ease the insertion.

Now here is a good tip for the best type of lube to use. Buy some Xylocaine or Lidocaine gel lubricant in a tube. They provide lubrication and contain a pain reliever to make insertion more comfortable. KY Jelly will also work if that is all you have.

Some Xylocaine brands come with a special cone applicator cap with a narrow tip that you can insert into the opening of your penis. Once inserted, you squeeze some lubricant into your penis opening. (You can do this with just the tip of the tube if it comes with no special applicator.) It will lubricate the catheter and act as a desensitizer so you barely feel the catheter going in. Just make sure the tube tip has been wiped with alcohol to make it sanitary. I go into this in detail later on.

Some catheters are pre-lubed, and they do not need any Xylocaine unless you feel extra lubrication is need. Yup, these are the catheters to use! Read on!

Lubricated Catheters

These types are relatively new and are the Rolls Royce of catheters because the lubrication makes them easy to insert! The whole catheter is lubricated. They just glide right in!

I was so pleased when I used these types of catheters the last few times I needed one. I wish I had had them before! They are worth the extra price. And they are fast to insert. That's why some are known as the brand "Speedicath."

Note: Some lubricated catheters come dry in the package and require you to insert a tablespoon or two of water to the open end of the package while it is held vertically. The water activates the lubrication in seconds. Know which type you are buying so this extra step does not surprise you in conditions where clean water is not available.

Touchless lubricated catheters are the best of them all as they are perfect for male catheter insertion. Unlike a permanent long-term catheter, these are single-use hydrophilic disposable catheters. "Hydrophylic" means they have a thin hydrophilic surface coating—and what a difference lubrication makes!

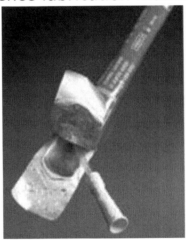

Individually packed and sterile, hydrophilic disposable catheters are the best of the best. As I said some are ready to use without the addition of water. They can be used right out of the package.

Others will require you to add the water first, which causes the coating to swell to a smooth, slippery film and makes the catheter far easier, safer and more comfortable to insert.

They can be inserted by just holding the opposite end from that which is inserted. That's why they are called "touchless"—you don't have to touch the tube itself. Without the special lubrication that makes them slide in so much easier, they could not be called "touchless."

The whole catheter is manipulated from the end you hold. Once the other tip is inserted, all you do is push gently and steadily to get it to go through into the bladder.

For prostate attacks and your emergency use, get the 12- or 14-gauge. They are quite thin. They are fast to use and basically require nothing else other than something to wash the tip of your penis—soap and water, or an alcohol or iodine wipe. And always have a 16-gauge one for backup because it will work just in case the narrower ones don't.

Catheter Tip Types:

There are two types of tips for lubricated and non-lubricated catheters:

- straight-tipped catheters, or
- Coudé catheters, which have a slight bend at the tip to allow easier passage through

an enlarged prostate. This angled part is only about ¼" long.

The best catheters have highly polished smooth tips to make insertion as easy as possible.

Coudé Catheters

My first choice is the SpeediCath Coudé Intermittent Catheters (bit.ly/r5qZev), as seen in the image. They make catheter insertion as simple and pain free as possible and are made for easy self-catheterization.

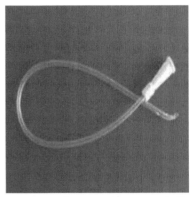

Coudé is French for "elbowed." This catheter is a special type of catheter for use by men especially if they have a prostate condition. An enlarged prostate makes catheter insertion trickier because of the pressure on the pee tube, or urethra.

Coudé catheters have a slight bend at the tip to allow easier passage through an enlarged prostate. This angled part is only about ¼" long.

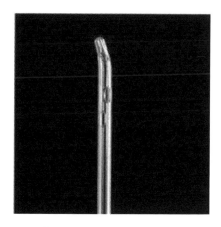

You can see the slight curve above.

Notice also the eyelets below the tip to allow the urine to enter the catheter. There are usually two of them. One on each side, offset by about a ½" or 1 cm.

Note: When you insert the catheter, it has to go past the entrance into the bladder so the eyelets are far enough inside the bladder for the urine to enter the eyelets (part of the reason the catheters are so long).

If you have BPH, or enlarged prostate conditions, then Coudé is the type of catheter to use. You can still get by with straight-tipped ones, but the help a Coudé catheter gives is worthwhile to use if you have a choice. Straight-tipped or Coudé—it is just a matter of personal preference.

A well-designed Coudé catheter will have a slight ridge or colored marking on the opposite end of the catheter, the part you hold. You can align it facing upwards so the tip is positioned correctly as it moves through your urethra to the prostate.

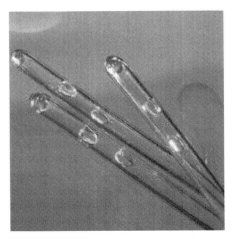

Coudé catheters are a bit more expensive than others, but the ease of application, for the hopefully rare occasions that you will have to use them, makes the price well worth it. They take the trauma and worry away—believe me—because I have had difficulties getting the cheap ones through the last inch or two on several occasions.

Be extremely careful when buying catheters and ensure they are sterile; sterility has been built into the package design of these SpeediCath beauties (bit.ly/r5qZev).

You can order them by the box, or scroll down for the option of buying one at a time to try them out. You can choose 12 FR, 14" length (12 FR means 12-gauge size). A 14 FR is fine as well (14 gauge), and get a 16 gauge FR one as your backup. You can buy one at a time, although buying a box of them is the best deal.

Please don't skimp here! I will share tips on the cheaper ones in case that is all you have, but these SpeediCaths (either Coudé or straight) are the ones to buy (bit.ly/r5qZev). Period.

Long-Term Catheters

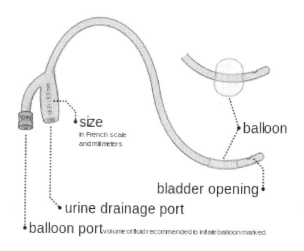

size
in French scale
and millimeters

balloon

bladder opening

urine drainage port

balloon port volume of fluid recommended to inflate balloon marked

Indwelling Foley Catheters

An indwelling Foley catheter is a type of catheter designed to stay inside your bladder for a period of time. As such, it is used after prostate cancer surgery, when your prostate blocks and you can't void your urine and if the doctor wants you to keep the catheter in for a while.

Catheters come in different shapes at both ends depending on their use. Long-term use requires that the inserted tip be held in place while inside the bladder and not be easily removed or dislodged while sleeping or moving.

This is done by being able to inflate a little balloon on the end that rests inside your bladder by pumping it up from the external end that has two openings, one for that function and one for the urine to exit.

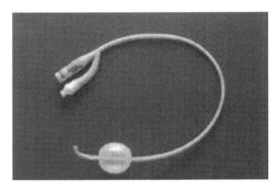

When inflated, the balloon keeps the Foley catheter securely in place so they can be worn for a longer period of time.

These Foley catheters are then attached to another flexible tube from the external end that goes to a plastic bag to collect the urine, holding about a liter or quart. The bag can be attached to a device beside the bed in a hospital or to your leg with a strap so you can walk around.

After prostate surgery, the indwelling Foley catheter is used so urine can flow while healing takes place. It is used for both prostate cancer surgery and enlarged prostate (BPH) surgery, such as TURP surgery in which part of the inside of the prostate is removed.

For surgical uses, the Foley catheters are probably at the thicker sizes—16 gauge and above—to allow blood to escape without clogging the tube. For most intermittent uses of a catheter, a 12 or 14 gauge is adequate and more comfortable to insert.

If you have had a Foley catheter put in place for an enlarged prostate that is blocked, please read up on what to do for a prostate attack, as discussed in my first chapter. It is often enough to just drain the bladder and then you can remove the catheter. The medical staff will usually want to leave it in place for days or weeks but, in my experience, this is overkill.

If you can find what triggered the prostate attack you can then avoid doing the same thing again—usually it is a food, supplement or drug like an antihistamine that is not positive for you. (See "What Triggers the Attack" in Chapter 1.)

I would remove the indwelling Foley catheter as soon as possible if it is in there for a prostate attack and not a surgery. If you do not believe that you can find out what triggered the reaction, then you will adapt to wearing the catheter and drain bag. I have found that 99% of the time, after removing the catheter, I am able to void well.

In the next chapter, I cover step-by-step instructions for insertion.

Chapter 3:
Exact Steps for Painless & Successful Self-Insertion

Male catheter insertion requires a precise series of steps so as to avoid pain if done properly.

Proper techniques will help you insert the catheter successfully even with an enlarged prostate. By following my steps, you will succeed and you will feel discomfort but not pain.

I have done it many times and have learned many simple tricks to ensure your success. Please read up on the causes of prostate problems in my book *Healthy Prostate: The Extensive Guide to Prevent and Heal Prostate Problems* so you can learn how to avoid this crisis in the future (www.healthyprostate.co/)!

Learning about catheters is an important first step so you can choose the best one to use. And even without the best ones, you will still succeed, saving you the time and hassle of going to a hospital if you have a sudden prostate attack that shuts you down.

But I want to make something clear to you, dear reader. I am not a doctor and cannot take responsibility for your decision to do self-catheterization, the term used to describe the do-it-yourself process of catheter insertion.

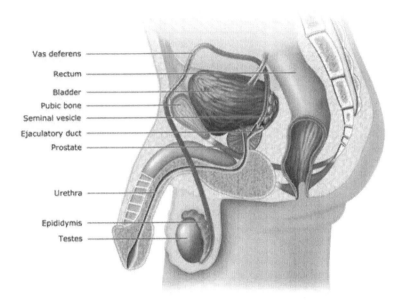

Vas deferens
Rectum
Bladder
Pubic bone
Seminal vesicle
Ejaculatory duct
Prostate
Urethra
Epididymis
Testes

Although many men insert their own catheters, it is a decision you should take in consultation with your medical professional. And if this is an emergency situation in which you cannot get to a doctor, then you will find my steps invaluable.

You see, I know because I had to do it many times with an extremely enlarged prostate, which blocks the last bit of the prostatic urethra and makes it more difficult to get the catheter through. The prostatic urethra is the part of the urethra pee tube that goes through the inside of your prostate (see diagram above).

Hey guys, you know all about the right tools for the job. The same applies here. Get the tools right and, with some good technique, you will be able to do this.

Self-Catheterization for Men

These modern internal male catheters have enabled men to have more freedom than ever before and to have peace of mind for emergencies where sudden blockage occurs. Be prepared if you have any symptoms of a prostate problem. Get a kit together so if an emergency happens, you can handle it safely. In fact, a catheter should be part of every first aid emergency kit today as well as the knowledge of how to use it.

How to Insert a Lubricated Internal Catheter

The first thing you'll have to do is acquire the necessary contents of you kit. The list below will help you with your purchases.

Lubricated Catheter Prostate Kit

Here is a list of items to create your minimal Prostate Kit. If you want less expensive catheters, go to this link for more information about other catheters (bit.ly/r5qZev).

Minimal Prostate Kit:

- one SpeediCath lubricated catheter: either a SpeediCath Intermittent Coudé

Catheter (bit.ly/r5qZev) or Straight-Tip SpeediCath (bit.ly/qiCGDF).

- a 12-gauge, 14″ (12 FR, 14" Length) catheter for men or a 14-gauge one (14 FR, 14" Length). Buy several so that you have backups for the car, home, work, travel bag, etc. FR stands for the gauge, which is the thickness of the tube. Even though 12 is thinner, the slightly thicker 14-gauge size may be optimum for its added help getting through the enlarged prostate.

- one 16-gauge catheter (16 FR) as an extra in the rare case that you experience difficulties with the thinner 12 FR or 14 FR one inserting the last bit through the prostate into the bladder.

- six to ten Alcohol Prep Pads: You can get 200 for a few bucks at this link (bit.ly/qaLEJ9).

- Xylocaine (optional): Xylocaine Ointment Tube (tiny.cc/ly26hx) *or* Lidocaine (tiny.cc/hqyu6). With SpeediCath (tiny.cc/o226hx), you really do not need this, but if you are worried at all about it hurting, then get some. Read the instructions on how to insert a non-lubricated catheter to know how to use the Xylocaine properly.

- a plastic Ziplock bag to hold all the items together as your emergency prostate kit.

For home use:

- the same kit as described above, but you can substitute a bottle of alcohol with Kleenex tissues that you wet for sterilizing in place of the Alcohol Prep Pads.
- include two towels to place under you on your bed.

Tip: Add a SpeediCath Coudé Intermittent Touchless Catheter to your first aid kit (bit.ly/r5qZev).

Advantages of lubricated catheters:

1. Self-contained unit lubricated and ready to go.
2. Much quicker and easier to use.
3. Not necessary to have anything else so easy to travel with and fast to use.
4. Much easier insertion because it is so slippery.
5. It costs more but is it ever worth the extra!
6. You can buy them individually or a box to save.

Some lubricated catheters require the addition of a tablespoon or two of water to actually lube them at the time you use them.

If you bought ones like that, and they are dry when you open the package, then just add a couple of tablespoons of water to the pack while holding it vertically and wait a minute or two for it to do its job. Make sure you know what type you have so you are prepared in advance. For travel, it would be best not to have to add water; therefore, you want a wet lubricated style. If you have a choice, always go with wet lubrication. Be prepared and buy the wet Speedicath lubricated catheters (bit.ly/r5qZev).

That's why I love the SpeediCaths because the lubrication on the whole tube is gentler on you—it is hyper-**slippery**. It makes male catheter insertion so much easier!

Coudé Catheter

In this section, I cover step-by-step instructions for how to insert a lubricated straight tip or Coudé catheter.

The only difference is the Coudé catheter has a line or ridge on the outside end of the catheter (the part you hold) to help guide it through with the angled internal tip facing upwards.

Inserting a lubricated catheter at home:

Note: What follows are very detailed steps. It is basically very simple: insert a tube slowly and gently through your penis making sure it is sterile at all times. The exact details follow.

1. Gather all the listed items in the minimal prostate kit discussed earlier in this chapter, which you should have ready in a kit in a Ziplock bag. Get 2 towels and a

plastic collection bottle for the urine: a liter or quart size is adequate.

2. Wash your hands really well then wash your penis with the glans pulled back if you are uncircumcised.

3. Decide where to do the job. I really prefer lying down leaning up on pillows, which is different from standing. Why? Because unlike regular users who use catheters every day (perhaps because of a spinal cord injury), you are in trauma by now, having tried everything, and still you can't release. You have an enlarged prostate problem and are experiencing pain. Lying down helps you relax and is less stressful than standing or even sitting (which is a good second choice). You do not have to be in the bathroom for this.

4. Lay a protective towel under you and another to the side where your bottle will be placed. This bottle will be where you put the external end of the catheter tube to collect the urine once it is inserted.

5. Place the items from the kit on the side towel.

6. Pull back the tab on the back of the catheter package to expose the sticky part. Attach the sticky part to the bedframe or side table within easy reach and pull down on the pull-tab enough to

expose the catheter top without touching anything inside.

7. Take the bottle of alcohol or alcohol wipes, remove the cap and pour some onto the Kleenex or open the swipe pads. You can also use iodine wipes if you prefer. The goal now is to sterilize everything. Always remember that what you touch from now on must be wiped clean before using. And you must re-wipe your fingers if you touch something not yet sterile! Be very careful so as to avoid the risk of possible infection through careless use.

8. Sterilize your hands and then the top of your penis with the glans pulled down using the alcohol pad or tissue. Wipe your hands again after as it just touched your penis.

9. One hand (your dominant one) now takes the catheter out of the package by gently taking the top of the exposed catheter, pulling it out of the package and, without touching the lower part of the catheter, guides the catheter tip into the opening at the tip of the penis while the other hand holds the penis with the glans down, tip opened and the penis vertical up from the body. Hold your penis up from your body with one hand so it is at a **RIGHT ANGLE** to your stomach.

10. If the catheter by accident touches anything, then wipe the spot with a clean tissue with alcohol on it. Then reinsert. Be hyper-careful at all times that what goes into the penis is sterile.

11. If using a Coudé catheter, notice that on the outside external tip of the Coudé catheter, a raised line shows you which way the Coudé tip is bent. Have that mark facing you upwards—that is the correct angle for it to help pass through the prostate. If using a straight catheter then this does not matter.

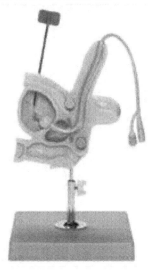

12. Once the catheter is in at the tip of the penis, steadily push it and it will glide its way through quite easily and with only minor discomfort.

13. Once inside, you start to push at a steady slow pace. **PULL YOUR PENIS UP STRONGLY SO IT IS STICKING STRAIGHT UP** at a **RIGHT ANGLE** to your body. STRETCHING IT WILL MAKE IT EASIER TO FIND ITS WAY THROUGH AS IT GOES DEEPER! **THIS IS AN IMPORTANT TECHNIQUE!**

    Notice that the penis is held up at a right angle to the body. This is important. If not, two bends would be **required** to insert it. Always insert with your penis held up at right angles!

14. Remember to breathe deeply and relax! You are almost done! Continue to push it through.

15. After 8–10 inches you will be coming to the bend at the entrance to the prostate and then through the prostate to the entrance to the bladder.

16. The sphincter muscle now has to relax enough to let the catheter through. If all goes well, it slips through into the bladder. If you feel any resistance, STOP pushing. Finesse is the key to success now and the smooth tip will be helping you out.

    Take your time to breathe deep and relax. Catheter insertion requires being gentle! The catheter may at this point be sliding back outwards a bit from its furthest point inside. Take some deep breaths and make a cough as you insert the catheter deeper. The sphincter muscle then can relax and release.

17. You basically want to knock on the door and give a bit of time for the sphincter to relax and open. Wait a few seconds. Cough and proceed.

18. Push gently. Never force. If it seems blocked and won't pass through, here is the trick to that—KEEP PULLING UP ON YOUR PENIS AND COUGH!

19. If need be, pull back and out a little bit (an inch or 2) and then start forward in again with a slight twisting motion back and forth. Cough again.

20. Ensure that the line is up as we mentioned above if using a Coudé type.

21. Twist the catheter with your fingers maybe a quarter of a turn or more, and that will help find a way through. Keep twisting back and forth and very gently pushing until it slips through the last little bit. Most of the time it will go through without any problem.

22. Finesse is the trick. **Never force it!**

23. FINESSE—GENTLE—TWIST and Cough. You will succeed easily with this trick (if you should need it). I didn't need it after I discovered the SpeediCath Coudé catheter. They are just so good! If at any

time you encounter resistance, pull back a bit and use the finesse turning trick and the cough to help the catheter through. ALWAYS KEEP PULLING STRONGLY UP ON YOUR PENIS!

24. Once you pop through into the bladder, push it far enough in so the eyelets can drain the urine (and it will seem like a lot of the catheter has disappeared inside— leaving 2–3 inches outside), suddenly urine will squirt free from the external end. Just put your thumb against the end and place it in the bottle. Then push the catheter a little further so that it is well inside the bladder.

    If you want, you can put your finger on the external tip before it enters the bladder, so as not to have the urine release into the air. Just place it in the bottle as you move it through the last bit. But hey! You will be so happy to see that squirt of urine—who cares at this point!

25. Keep the bottle with the external end of the catheter inside it as low as you can beside you so gravity works to void the bladder. You can stop pulling up on your penis now!

26. You should now be emptying and feeling such a wonderful sense of relief. Aaaah! Oh so good! At last relief! Such an

immediate feeling of relief and well-being washes over you!

27. Job well done! Keep holding the catheter in place so that it doesn't slip out a bit.

28. Just lie there and feel the blessings of this little device that just saved your life!

29. The bottle will be receiving more and more of the urine, slowing down eventually to a trickle after a few minutes.

30. Relax and empty. Oh feels so good now!

31. After a few minutes or so—there is no rush—and no more urine flows, then slowly remove a bit of the catheter towards the neck of the bladder. That may release the last bit of urine near the neck of the bladder.

32. When done, pull the catheter all the way out and discard beside you.

33. Rest a bit before clean up.

34. Sleep if you can.

35. There is no need to worry now, because the act of putting the catheter through seems to open the channel and keeps it open after it is out. Soon, you will have your first pee. It may burn a bit as the ammonia in the urine touches any part that may have been irritated by the catheter but this should be very minor as these are such good catheters. Any

discomfort will soon pass as the day progresses.

36. If you do not know the cause, do your detective work and figure out what caused the prostate attack. Now is the time to personally test all that you recently ate.

It is really quite easy to use a lubricated catheter, even though I have gone into great length to describe what to do. You can use them anywhere you have to. I always travel with one or two and some alcohol wipes, especially when traveling by air.

IMPORTANT! In the very rare case that your 12 FR or 14 FR catheter is unable to pass through the prostate using all the above techniques, then use the backup 16 FR one. Because it is wider, it will find its way better. The thinner ones are easier to use and for most people most of the time they work just fine. But it is nice to have a backup Plan B with the 16s.

During the day, you may feel a burning sensation as you pee due to irritation. The ammonia in your urine causes that feeling, but the ammonia is also sterilizing as the urine passes through. This burning will lessen and will pass in a day or so.

Note: It is possible over the next while (days to weeks) to pass some blood and blood-colored urine or even clots of blood from possible trauma of using the catheter or debris from the prostate. This condition will pass and is not cause for alarm unless you get steady amounts of fresh blood, which is a serious concern. Then seek medical help. Steady amounts of fresh blood should not result from regular use of a catheter.

After my first blockage requiring my doctor to insert a Foley catheter, I went to see a specialist: a urologist. He was a very busy doctor with many patients waiting and, knowing what I know now, he was a brute. He put a prostate–bladder camera up me without any local anesthesia. Was that ever painful!

He proceeded to put a new Foley catheter back inside me so he could dismiss me. Having worked as a teen with my father, an old-school compounding pharmacist, I was very well versed and meticulous about being sterile at all times when handling medications.

So, here was this doctor about to insert a catheter into me. I watched him. I was still in pain and shock from the camera job. He was wearing sterile gloves, but he made a mistake. I was too distressed to call him on it.

He tore open the new catheter package with his sterile gloves and took out the sterile catheter. Of course, the package itself was NOT sterile as I had had to purchase it elsewhere and bring it to the appointment! With his now 'unsterile' gloves, he grabbed the catheter with his dirty hands and inserted it into me! I was too shocked and in pain to call him to task!

I tell you this story so you can be smarter. Always ensure that you are sterile and that the last thing you touch before inserting your catheter is also sterile. That way, you will never have any problems with doing your own catheterization.

How to Insert Non-Lubricated Internal Catheters

The first thing you'll have to do is acquire the necessary contents of you kit. The list below will help you with your purchases.

Non-Lubricated Catheter Prostate Kit

Use a non-lubricated catheter like these excellent ones (tiny.cc/s826hx). Your choice of Straight or Coudé tip.

- a 12-gauge, 14" (12 FR, 14" Length) catheter for men or a 14-gauge one (14 FR, 14" Length). Buy several so that you have backups for the car, home, work, travel bag, etc. FR stands for the gauge, which is the thickness of the tube. Even though 12 is thinner the slightly thicker 14 gauge size may be optimum for its added help getting through the enlarged prostate.

- one 16-gauge catheter (16 FR) as an extra in the rare case that you experience difficulties with the thinner 12 FR or 14 FR one inserting the last bit through the prostate into the bladder.
- six to ten Alcohol Prep Pads: You can get 200 for a few bucks (bit.ly/qaLEJ9).
- Xylocaine: Xylocaine Ointment Tube (tiny.cc/ly26hx) or Lidocaine (tiny.cc/hqyu6) as a lubricant and desensitizer. In a pinch, you can use KY Jelly, but it has no desensitizer.
- a plastic Ziplock bag to hold all the items together as your emergency prostate kit.

For home use:

- the same kit as described above, but you can substitute a bottle of alcohol with Kleenex tissues that you wet for sterilizing in place of the Alcohol Prep Pads.
- include two towels to place under you on your bed.

Ensure that the sterility of all tools is maintained at all times. The urethra and bladder are naturally sterile areas. The penis must be properly cleansed before catheter insertion.

You will need to be more careful with sterility because more handling is involved than with lubricated catheters. Be meticulous to avoid infection. In all my many uses of self-catheterization, I have never had a urinary tract infection problem because I was always careful to keep everything sterile: hands and tools.

1. Gather all the listed items in the minimal prostate kit discussed earlier in this chapter, which you should have ready in a kit in a Ziplock bag. Get 2 towels and a plastic collection bottle for the urine: a liter or quart size is adequate.

2. Wash your hands really well then wash your penis with the glans pulled back if you are uncircumcised.

3. Decide where to do the job. I really prefer lying down leaning up on pillows. Why? Because unlike regular users who use catheters every day (perhaps because of a spinal cord injury), you are in trauma by now, having tried everything, and still you can't release. You have an enlarged prostate problem. Lying down helps you relax and is less stressful than standing or even sitting (which is a good second choice). You do not have to be in the bathroom for this.

4. Lay a protective towel under you and another to the side where your bottle will be to place the external end of the catheter tube to collect the urine.

5. Place the items from the kit on the side towel.

6. Lie down with your kit beside you. Hopefully you will have Xylocaine as a lubricant with desensitizer or another lubricant like KY Jelly if the other can't be had—but always a water-soluble one, never an oil-base lubricant like Vaseline. Vaseline may block the eyelet drain holes near the tip of the catheter and prevent or slow the urine coming out!

7. Take the bottle of alcohol or alcohol wipes, remove the cap and pour some onto the Kleenex or open the swipe pads. You can also use iodine wipes if you prefer. The goal now is to sterilize everything. Always remember that what you touch from now on must be wiped clean before using. And you must re-wipe your fingers if you touch something not yet sterile! Be very careful so as to avoid the risk of possible infection through careless use. Sterilize everything—the tube, the cap, the penis. I use several pieces of Kleenex with alcohol as I do all this.

8. Remove the catheter from the package by touching only the external end of the catheter. The outside package is not sterile so discard it, and keep it away from sterile areas.

9. Wipe your fingers again with alcohol; then wipe the catheter with alcohol and

place it on several flat pieces of Kleenex beside you.

10. Before using the KY or Xylocaine tube, wipe it first with alcohol and then open it. If there is a special applicator tip, wipe it and screw it on the tip of the tube with your sterile fingers. If not, then wipe the tip of the tube really well with alcohol.

    Being meticulously sterile with everything you touch is important.

11. Sterilize your hands and then the top of your penis with the glans pulled down using the pad or tissue. Wipe your hands again after since it just touched your penis.

12. Hold your penis with one hand up from your body so it is at a **RIGHT ANGLE** to your stomach. Pull back the glans and open the tip of the penis.

13. Insert the tip of the lubrication tube and give a good squeeze of lubricant or Xylocaine into the penis.

14. Wipe the tube and its tip again for reuse. Wipe fingers again. Always wipe with fresh alcohol on tissue. Always remember to keep everything sterile.

15. Grab the catheter and wipe that again at the tip area up towards the external end.

16. Then apply generously some lubricant or Xylocaine to the catheter tip up to maybe

3–4 inches. Again, never use Vaseline—it is oil based and it could block the eyelit openings for urine entry into the catheter.

17. Now you are ready to insert the catheter into the tip of the penis making sure not to touch the catheter to anything but the entry into the penis. Be hyper-careful at all times that what goes into the penis is sterile.

    If the catheter by accident touches anything, then wipe the spot with a clean tissue with alcohol on it. Then reinsert. Be hyper-careful at all times that what goes into the penis is sterile.

18. If using a Coudé catheter, notice that on the outside external tip of the Coudé catheter, a raised line shows you which way the Coudé tip is bent. Have that mark facing you upwards—that is the correct angle for it to help pass through the prostate. If using a straight catheter then this does not matter.

19. Once inside, you start to push it in gently but at a steady slow pace. **PULL YOUR PENIS UP STRONGLY** so it is STICKING STRAIGHT UP at a right angle to your body. STRETCHING it will make it easier to find its way through as it goes deeper! This is an IMPORTANT TECHNIQUE! **PULL** your penis!

Notice that the penis is held up at a right angle to the body. This is important. If not, two bends would be **required** to insert it. Always insert with your penis held up at right angles!

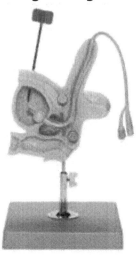

20. You can wipe the tube after the first few inches with Kleenex and alcohol to make sure it is sterile as you push it through and can add some more lubricant or Xylocaine if you want. But you are probably OK just to keep steadily pushing in. You can hold the end of the catheter or the catheter tube itself. If it is the tube just make sure that you are sterile before it enters.

21. Go gently but steadily, twisting it slightly as you do so. If there is any spot where it does not want to go further, then do NOT push hard! Instead use finesse to twist

the catheter until it can find a way through. FINESSE—GENTLE—TWIST. Pay attention please!!! If you still find it hard to get through, it is because your prostate is really inflamed and enlarged.

If you are using a Coudé tip catheter then ensure that the marking is facing upwards towards you... this helps it find its way.

22. Take your time to breathe deep and relax. Catheter insertion requires being gentle! The catheter may at this point be sliding back outwards from its furthest point inside. Take some deep breaths and make a cough as you insert the catheter deeper. The sphincter muscle then can relax and release.

23. Just twist it a bit and start moving it deeper in. ALWAYS KEEP PULLING STRONGLY UP ON YOUR PENIS! With gentle finesse, it will find a way through. Just be patient until it pushes through. But never ever force it. Just twist a bit and gently push. Back off if you need to and move it gently back with a slight twist, and you will succeed. Always pull your penis up as described above. Sometimes it is like knocking on the door so the sphincter can relax and open.

Remember to breathe deeply and relax! You are almost done! Continue to push it through.

24. After 8–10 inches you will be coming to the bend at the entrance to the prostate and then through the prostate to the entrance to the bladder.

25. The sphincter muscle now has to relax enough to let the catheter through. If all goes well, it slips through into the bladder. If you feel any resistance, STOP pushing. Finesse is the key to success now and the smooth tip will be helping you out.

    Take your time to breathe deep and relax. Catheter insertion requires being gentle! The catheter may at this point be sliding back outwards a bit from its furthest point inside. Take some deep breaths and make a cough as you insert the catheter deeper. The sphincter muscle then can relax and release.

26. You basically want to knock on the door and give a bit of time for the sphincter to relax and open. Wait a few seconds. Cough and proceed.

27. Push gently. Never force. If it seems blocked and won't pass through, here is the trick to that—KEEP PULLING UP ON YOUR PENIS and cough!

28. If need be, pull back and out a little bit (an inch or 2) and then start forward in again with a slight twisting motion back and forth. Cough again.

29. As we mentioned above, ensure that the line is up if you're using a Coudé type.

30. Twist the catheter with your fingers, maybe a quarter of a turn or more, and that will help find a way through. Keep twisting back and forth and very gently pushing until it slips through the last little bit. Most of the time it will go through without any problem.

31. Finesse is the trick. Never force it!

32. FINESSE—GENTLE—TWIST and Cough. You will succeed easily with this trick (if you should need it). If at any time you encounter resistance, pull back a bit and use the finesse turning trick and the cough to help the catheter through. ALWAYS KEEP PULLING STRONGLY UP ON YOUR PENIS!

33. Once you pop through into the bladder, push it far enough in so the eyelets can drain the urine. (It will seem like a lot of the catheter has disappeared inside—leaving 2–3 inches outside.) Suddenly urine will squirt free from the external end. Just put your thumb against the end and place it in the bottle. Then push the

catheter a little further so that it is well inside the bladder.

If you want, you can put your finger on the external tip before it enters the bladder, so as not to have the urine release into the air. Just place it in the bottle as you move it through the last bit. But hey! You will be so happy to see that squirt of urine—who cares at this point!

34. Keep the bottle as low as you can beside you so gravity works to void the bladder. You can stop pulling up on your penis now!

35. You should now be emptying and feeling such a wonderful sense of relief. Aaaah! Oh so good! At last relief!

36. Job well done! Keep holding the catheter in place so that it doesn't slip out a bit.

37. Just lie there and feel the blessings of this little device that just saved your life!

38. The bottle will be receiving more and more of the urine, slowing down eventually to a trickle after a few minutes.

39. Relax and empty. Oh, feels so good now!

40. After a few minutes or so—there is no rush—and no more urine flows, then slowly remove a bit of the catheter (about 1" or 2 cm). That may release the last bit of urine near the neck of the bladder.

41. When done, pull the catheter all the way out and discard beside you.
42. Rest a bit before clean up.
43. Sleep if you can.
44. There is no need to worry now because the act of putting the catheter through seems to open the channel and keeps it open after it is out. Soon, you will have your first pee. It may burn a bit as the ammonia in the urine touches any part that may have been irritated by the catheter. Any discomfort will soon pass as the day progresses.
45. If you do not know the cause, do your detective work and figure out what caused the prostate attack. Now is the time to personally test all that you recently ate.

IMPORTANT! In the very rare case that your 12 FR or 14 FR catheter is unable to pass through the prostate using all the above techniques, then use the backup 16 FR one. Because it is wider, it will find its way better. The thinner ones are easier to use and, for most people, most of the time they work just fine. But it is nice to have a backup Plan B with the 16s.

During the day, you may feel a burning sensation as you pee due to irritation. The ammonia in your urine causes that feeling, but the ammonia is also sterilizing as the urine passes through. This burning will lessen and will pass in a day or so.

Note: It is possible over the next while (days to weeks) to pass some blood and blood-colored urine or even clots of blood from possible trauma of using the catheter or debris from the prostate. This condition will pass and is not cause for alarm unless you get steady amounts of fresh blood, which is a serious concern. Then seek medical help. Steady amounts of fresh blood should not result from regular use of a catheter.

Note: If you use a non-lubricated Coudé catheter with the elbow tip, then the only addition to the above instructions is to notice the little edge line on the external end of the catheter that you hold. Turn this up so you can see it.

That positions the Coudé end to be upwards helping to find its way through the prostatic urethra (the tube that goes through your prostate). You can still twist back and forth a bit if needed to assist but, in general, the alignment is upwards.

Catheter Insertion Away from Home

If you are on the road and have a prostate blockage, hopefully you have your kit with you. Find a washroom. Grab some paper towels and enter a stall. I have found it best to sit on the toilet rather than stand. Pants down. Paper towels on lap. Kit placed on top. Then follow the steps to insert.

The difference is that you need to be **extremely** careful about being sterile in a public washroom. Your penis will be up and away from the toilet so that helps. The toilet bowl becomes your 'bottle' once the catheter is all the way in. Remember the thumb on end trick just as you push through into the bladder. This way you can avoid getting urine on you as you direct the end of the tube into the toilet bowl.

I have done this at an airport, in the airplane, and in hotels. Just be careful and hyper clean, and you will be fine for this kind of an emergency.

How to Avoid Catheter Problems

Here are ways that can help you avoid catheter problems:

1. Choose the right kind: male catheters.
2. Choose the right gauge: the ideal for one-time use is 12s and 14s. These are quite thin and far less painful than you imagine. In fact, a better word to use is "discomfort" and not painful. You will sing its praises once the urine exits!

    Sometimes a larger catheter is necessary for successful insertion, contrary to intuition. The reason for this is because a larger catheter is stiffer and, therefore, can provide a bit more force to open the prostatic urethra. That is why it is good to have the 16 gauge as a backup.

3.   Choose a single use catheter (also known as short-term or intermittent catheters)— they are removed after you have emptied your bladder.

4.   Use the right kind of catheter tip. For an enlarged prostate, use a Coudé catheter. The tip has a slight bend to make it easier to go through the prostate. But straight ones work fine, too.

5.   For problems with dribbling, urgency and frequency when not at home, use an external male catheter.

Reusing Catheters

It is possible to save money by reusing a catheter. But please do the following:

1.   Do not try to reuse and clean a lubricated catheter. Just non-lubricated ones are possible.

2.   Rinse clean under warm water.

3.   Either (a) add hot water to a bowl and a ¼ cup of vinegar and let soak for a couple of hours, or (b) boil in a pot of water for 5 minutes.

4. After cooling if boiled or rinsed in hot water to remove the vinegar, put on a paper towel to dry.
5. After it is dry on the outside, take the external end of the catheter and swing in a circle to help remove any moisture inside the tube and then let completely dry
6. Put in a zip lock bag for reuse.

External Catheters or Male Condom Catheters

External male catheters are used for occasions in which you know you may have troubles finding or getting to a bathroom, or do not want to be interrupted by frequent or urgent urination. Truck and taxi drivers, long-distance travel, sports events, and other occasions are just some possible users or uses of these wonderful devices.

External catheter = Going. Can't Stop.

They go over your penis like a condom and have a tube at the end to drain into a bag. The trick is to keep them from falling off or getting loose because if they do, they'll leak or won't work properly.

Size Matters! This is where an honest measurement of your favorite part must be accurate! Cheat and call it longer or thicker and you will leak! If the external catheter is too small, it may hurt during the time you're wearing it. Go here to download a sizing chart: Merlin Medical Supply Sizing Chart (tiny.cc/cx36hx).

Now that you know what the right size is for you, I will explain how an external male catheter works and help you choose what kind to buy.

You have several choices of external condom catheters, all of which attach to a drainage bag with a tube. They come in rubber, polyvinyl or silicone. They're attached by double-sided adhesive, a latex inflatable cuff, jockey's type strap or foam strap. They're disposable and really shouldn't be used for more than 24–48 hours. Reusable ones are available.

Always remember that with any catheter a risk of infection exists. Even external catheters can cause skin irritation; an adhesive belt inside the condom part sticks to the skin of the penis and wraps around it holding it in place.

For more information about Managing Urinary Incontinence with Catheters, visit tiny.cc/e136hx

Different men have different levels of activity. Therefore, urinary drainage storage bags come in various sizes. For example, men who are still active can get a smaller bag.

Want to read more about them?

- What is a Condom Catheter? (tiny.cc/r336hx)

- How to Care For Your Condom Catheter (tiny.cc/t436hx)

As you have read, there are many types of external male catheters. You will have to read more and explore your options to find ones that work best for you. The best idea is to try several types and see what works for you.

- Sources of External Condom Catheters:
- Top of the Line External Catheter (tiny.cc/z836hx)
- Best seller & inexpensive external catheter #1 (bit.ly/oaKjsB)
- Best seller & inexpensive external catheter #2 (bit.ly/nYIypQ)

Search for other brands: put *condom catheters* into the search field: Search (bit.ly/oOeANx)

External Condom Catheters

These can be useful for those occasions when you know access to a bathroom will be limited, but you know that you will have to go frequently. Just get one of these to ease your worries.

Here are step-by-step instructions for using external condom catheters:

1. First, wash your hands.
2. Next, gather your supplies: correct-sized condom catheter, leg-drainage bag with

tubing, clamp, manicure scissors, soap, wash cloth, towel and protective ointment.

3. Use the manicure scissors to cut back the hair at the base of the penis. This prevents it from being caught by the adhesive.

4. Remember, the penis and surrounding area must be cleansed thoroughly with soap and water. Dry completely before applying a new catheter. This is crucial because if moisture is left inside the condom, bacteria can grow. Bacteria can cause a urinary tract infection. You don't need that on top of your prostate problem!

5. Sometimes, you might find the adhesive used inside the condom catheter causes irritation to the skin on the shaft of the penis. In this case, avoid using the condom catheter until the irritation is gone.

6. Urine can irritate the skin, so use a protective ointment, such as zinc oxide, and let it dry before attaching your condom catheter.

7. Tightly roll the balloon-like part, the condom sheath, to the edge of the connector tip. Next, put the catheter sheath on the end of your penis, but leave

about 1/2" space between the two tips: the penis tip and the connector tip.

8. It's easiest if you let your penis stretch as you unroll the condom smoothly. When done, gently press it to the penis so it sticks.

9. Connect the tip to the tube to the urine bag and strap the bag to your thigh.

10. For removal, clamp the tube closed to prevent spillage. Disconnect the tubing, unstrap the bag and remove the condom by rolling it forward. Then empty the pee bag.

This video demonstrates the application of an external condom catheter (tiny.cc/dg46hx). Good to have as a backup.

Conclusion

Men are unlucky today to have so many prostate problems.

But we are ever so lucky to have such wonderful catheters for those cases in which we need them. Be prepared in advance. For emergencies, have a prostate kit on hand and this booklet to explain how to use them.

By following the advice in this book, you can save yourself a lot of grief and money. Use your doctor and emergency department in a crisis, and follow this advice in those cases where you need a Plan B. Have the tools at hand, and you will discover that male catheter insertion can be done by you when needed.

Information for Professionals: Tips to Enable Successful Catheter Insertion

These techniques are more advanced but can help a nursing professional in difficult cases.

First ensure you have tried with a 16-gauge catheter. If that doesn't work, try one of these two techniques:

1. You can really lubricate the urethra well by filling a 30–50 mL sterile catheter-tipped syringe with a lubricant—ideally Xylocaine. Then inject it into the urethra with gentle pressure until the urethra can't take any more. Then insert the catheter. It should be a really well lubed tube now and will make it far easier to succeed with your 16-gauge catheter

2. Inject the lubricant into the catheter while the catheter is being passed slowly through the urethra. Fill the syringe as outlined above. Then insert the tip into the external end of the catheter and fill the catheter with a lubricant, such as Xylocaine ideally. As the catheter is being passed, slowly inject more lubricant to

ensure that the entire exterior length of the catheter is lubricated and to help dilate the urethra just ahead of the catheter tip as the lube is pushed out of the eyelets into the urethra.

In case the techniques described here do not work—including using a stiffer catheter with lots of lube and bigger size—then here are advanced medical techniques you can use:

- A Novel Technique for Difficult Male Urethral Catheterization (tiny.cc/1i46hx)
- Glidewire-Assisted Foley Catheter Placement: A Simple and Safe Technique for Difficult Male Catheterization (tiny.cc/pk46hx)

Here is a nursing educational video of how to insert a male catheter (tiny.cc/a146hx). It is very basic. It does not give any tips on how to deal with any insertion problems. And I would recommend for patient comfort the use of Xylocaine rather than just the gel as shown. For a bit extra cost, you can provide a much less difficult experience for the traumatized man lying on the bed!

If you enjoyed reading this book, I'd appreciate it if you would take a couple of minutes to post a short review at Amazon.

Intelligent reviews help other customers make better buying choices. And because I read all my reviews personally, they will help me to write better books in the future. Thanks for your support!

Ron Bazar

About the Author

Ronald M. Bazar, a Harvard MBA, is a health enthusiast and author of the new comprehensive book on the prostate called *Healthy Prostate: The Extensive Guide to Prevent and Heal Prostate Problems Including Prostate Cancer, BPH Enlarged Prostate and Prostatitis* which is available on Amazon, iTunes, Kindle and more outlets.

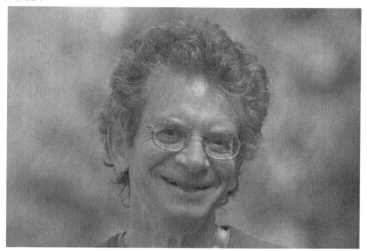

Ron, a "bit sweaty" after playing a long Ultimate Frisbee game at age 65!

Other Books by Ronald M. Bazar

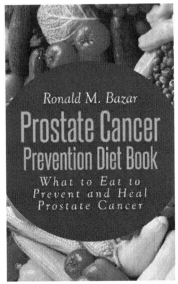

Prostate Cancer Prevention Diet

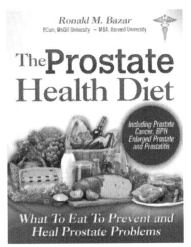

The Prostate Health Diet

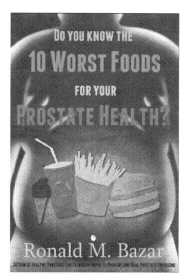

Do You Know the 10 Worst Foods for Your
Prostate Health?

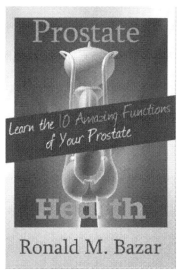

Prostate Health: Learn the 10 Functions of Your
Prostate

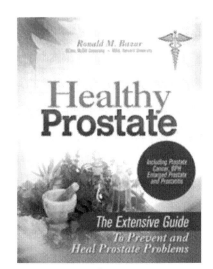

Healthy Prostate: The Extensive Guide to Prevent and Heal Prostate Problems Including Prostate Cancer, BPH Enlarged Prostate and Prostatitis

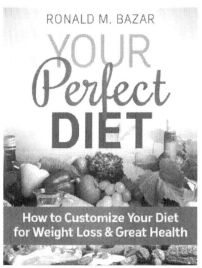

Your Perfect Diet

Other Unrelated Books:

BeaBea: Her Diary Her Life: Beatrice Millman Bazar: Her diary from the summer of 1931 and highlights from the rest of her life (with Kaima Bazar) (tiny.cc/bdnzzw)

Good Planets are Hard to Find (with Roma Dehr) (tiny.cc/9dnzzw)

From A to Z by Bike (with Roma Dehr) (tiny.cc/4enzzw)

I Love Not Smoking: An Activity Book for Non Smoking Children (with Roma Dehr) (tiny.cc/tfnzzw)

Websites

www.HealthyProstate.co

www.NaturalProstate.com

www.ArbutusArts.com
(my hobby business unrelated to prostate issues)

Made in the USA
San Bernardino, CA
09 September 2017